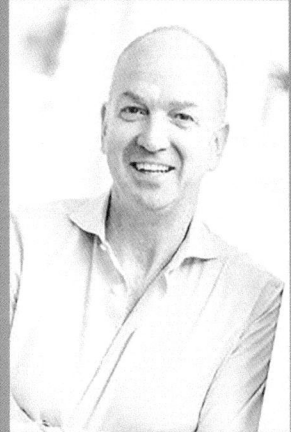

DR NEIL COUNIHAN

Dr Neil Counihan has been a non-executive director for an international stem cell biobank, and is an expert in storing stem cells from deciduous teeth. The UK's leading orthodontist and children's dental expert, he is the founder of several award-winning clinics and has lived in New York, Sydney, Mexico City and London, where he resides today with his two children, Callum, a medical student, and Lolly, a ski instructor. Dr Counihan's insatiable thirst for adventure has taken him from charitable organisations in Peru, to dirt biking in India, to extreme arctic marathons in Norway. When he's not aiming to make stem cells available to the wider public for life-saving treatments, you'll find him training to take on Grand Paradiso.

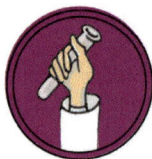

CHAPTERS

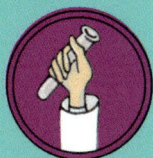

A NEW ERA OF MEDICINE

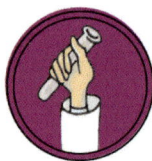

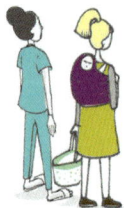

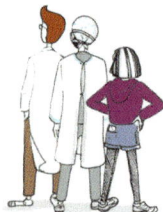

STOP

WHATEVER YOU'RE DOING
-RIGHT NOW-

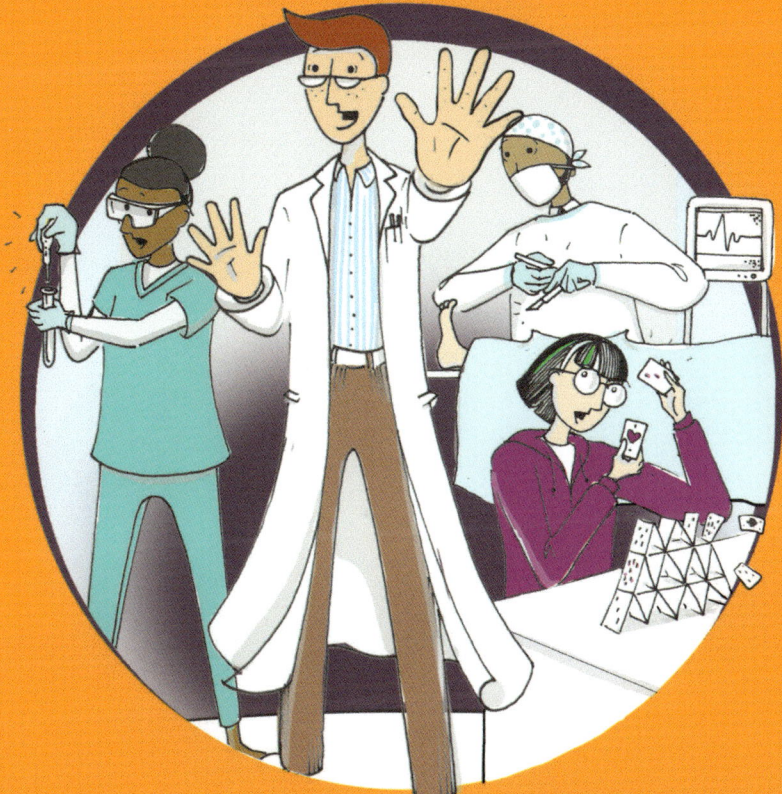

AND PICTURE THIS:

A world where we are not
dependent on pharmaceuticals

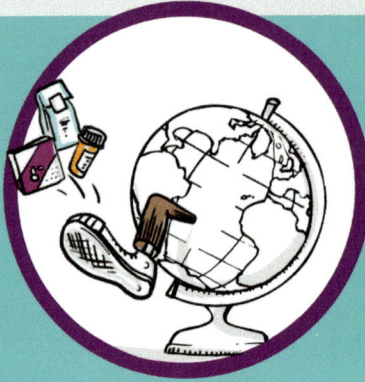

Where waiting time for
life-saving operations doesn't exist

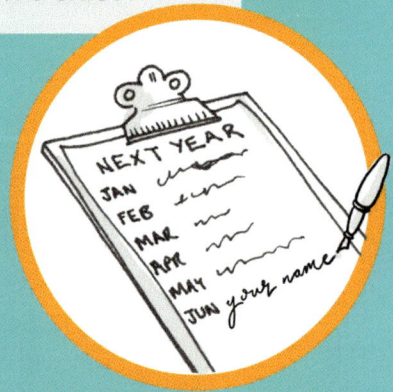

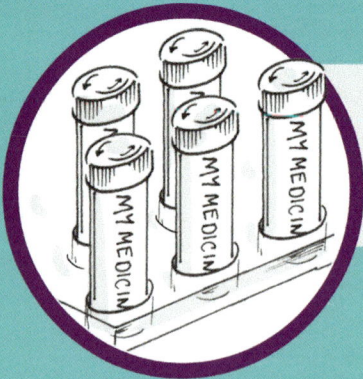

Where individually personalised
medicine is available to everyone.

Now imagine we told you that this is within our reach - that you, your children, and your grandchildren are living in an era which is going through this ground-breaking shift in medicine

right now.

Sound wacky? Well it's not - in fact, it's rather clever. We're talking about regenerative medicine, and here's what you need to know.

REGENERATIVE MEDICINE REFERS TO A BRANCH OF MEDICINE THAT USES THE BODY'S OWN NATURAL RESOURCES - ITS STEM CELLS - TO REPAIR, REBUILD AND RECOVER AFTER ILLNESS AND INJURY.

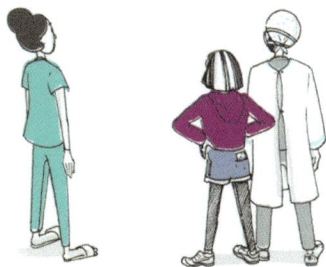

It is a drug-free solution; an ingeniously simple way of saving human lives - as well as enhancing the quality of those same lives in later years.

It has the power to change our healthcare industry forever - and for the better.

It is our **eureka** moment, our **future**, and our **right** as human beings.

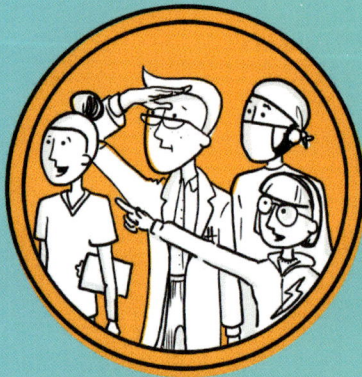

Only one question remains:

ARE YOU READY FOR IT?

2

THE STORY SO FAR

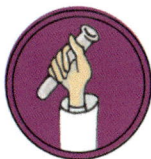

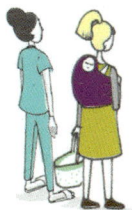

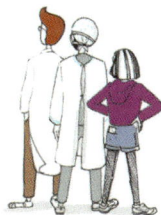

Of course, there's a lot of controversy surrounding stem cells. Right now, you're probably picturing a scientist in a white lab coat...

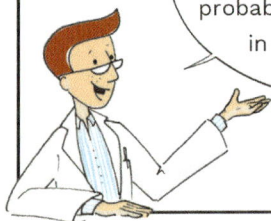

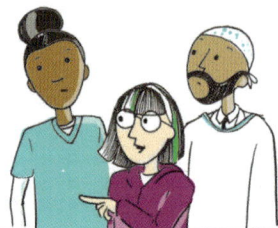

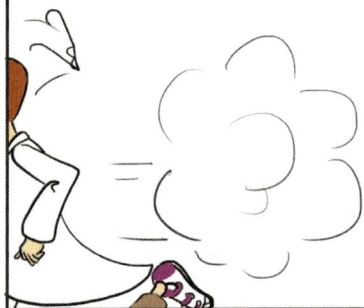

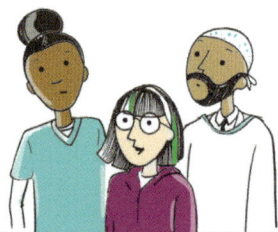

...a sort of modern-day Dr Frankenstein, working furiously to create a genetically superior creature in a test tube.

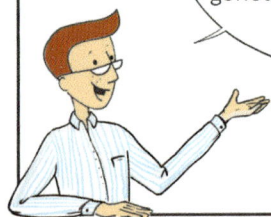

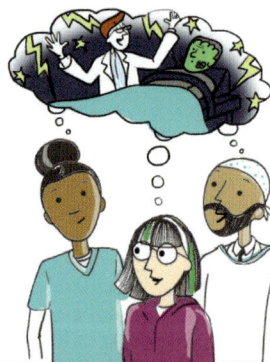

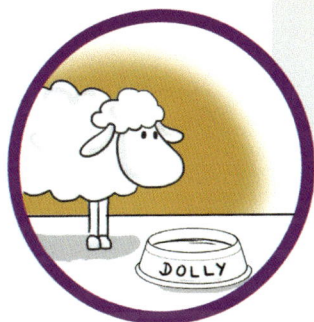

The case of Dolly the Sheep in 1996

- the world's first cloning experiment -

didn't help.

Dolly, now the world's most famous sheep, suffered from accelerated ageing and multiple organ failure, and the experiment was short-lived.

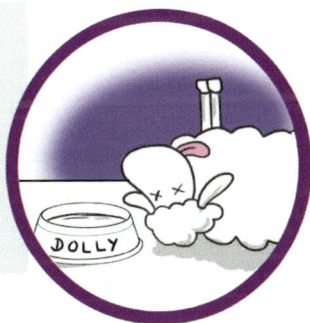

But through their attempts at recreating a natural species, scientists gained an incredible understanding of how cells do (and more importantly) DON'T work.

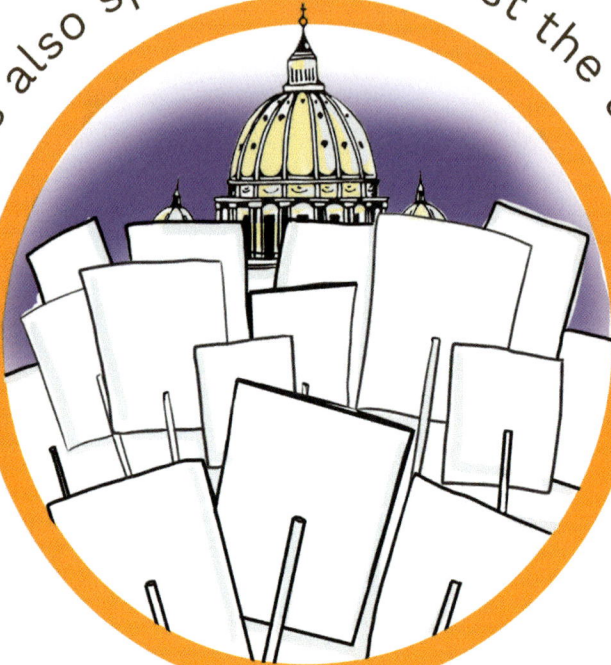

Religious groups also spoke out against the use of stem cells

A human life, they insisted, begins as a ball of cells. By taking those cells, you destroy the foetus that is developing. Which of course makes perfect sense.

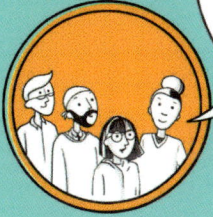

What you need to remember however, is that we're not talking about *embryonic* stem cells (stem cells harvested from a young human embryo), we're talking about *adult* stem cells.

Adult stem cells are found in cord blood, cord tissue and placenta - however, they are considered 'clinical waste', so they are routinely incinerated. Yet these 'waste products' are a safe and responsible source of stem cells.

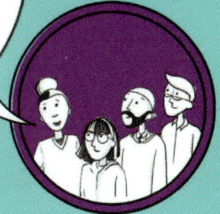

That last sentence isn't meant to make you squirm, it's meant to reassure you:

ADULT STEM CELLS
- LIKE SOLAR PANELS AND WIND TURBINES -
ARE SUSTAINABLE.

Thanks to the pioneering work of scientists and universities, our knowledge of stem cells has grown exponentially.

Today, they are used to treat 82 diseases - from leukaemia to sickle cell anaemia. Current trials and treatments include Type 1 diabetes, spinal cord injury, heart attacks and strokes.

The general public may slowly be coming around to the future of our healthcare, but regenerative medicine is still some way off becoming mainstream.

THIS NEEDS TO CHANGE.

3

THE BUILDING BLOCKS OF LIFE

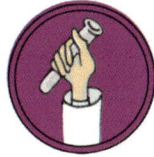

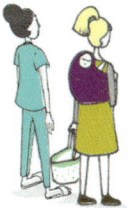

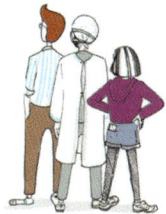

So let's get down to the nitty gritty. What exactly *are* stem cells anyway?

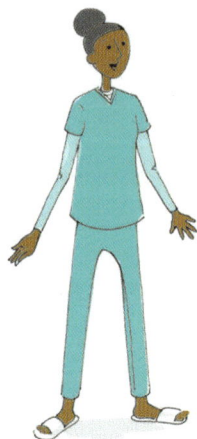

A human being (such as yourself) is a collection of 30 trillion cells - these make up every organ, every system and every biological structure in the body.

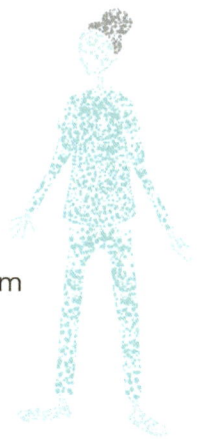

stem cells, however, are the

SUPERCHARGED

version

They are the only specialised cell in the

WHOLE ENTIRE BODY,

which not only makes them

mind-blowingly clever,

but means that they have a

unique ability to morph, or

'differentiate', into

any type of cell that they choose

- from BONE to TISSUE to CARTILAGE to ORGAN.

It's why they're referred to as the

'building blocks of life'.

TRY THIS.

Think of your body as a very clever, complex machine (which it is) - one that relies on hundreds of thousands of little cogs to run smoothly.

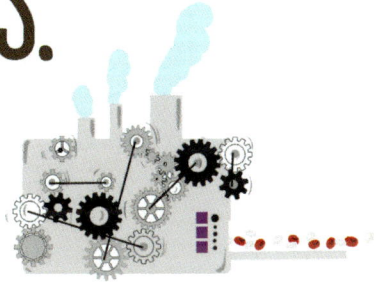

Of course, every once in a while, one of these cogs might get stuck, or irreparably broken. It happens.

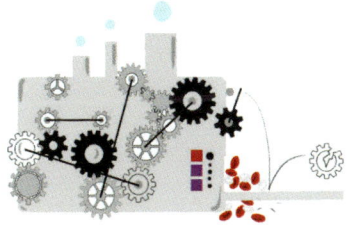

What the body needs NOW is a replacement cog. A cog that instinctively knows how the body works, and what role it plays in the machine.

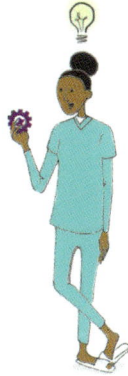

And this is where stem cells come in.

Once in place, the stem cell assumes it's new guise and starts to function as a brand-new cog. The body carries on as normal, the machine works as a whole once more. Neat, huh?

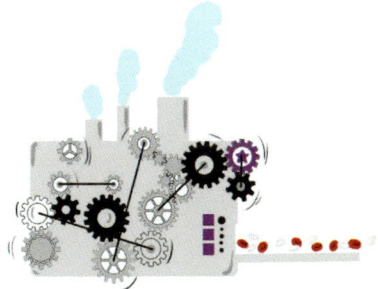

4

SO WHERE ARE THEY HIDING?

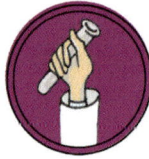

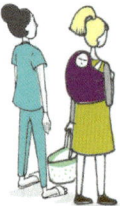

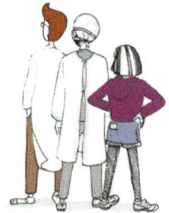

This is all good
and well.
But these
specialised cells
haven't always
been easy
to find.

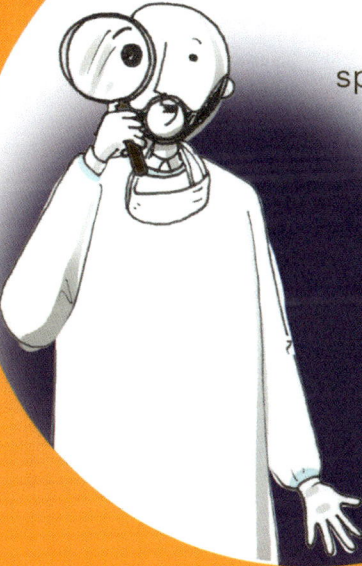

Bone Marrow is the most common source - but it's a lengthy, painful and invasive process, involving the donor undergoing a general anaesthetic in order for the extraction to be made (as a result, many donors change their mind).

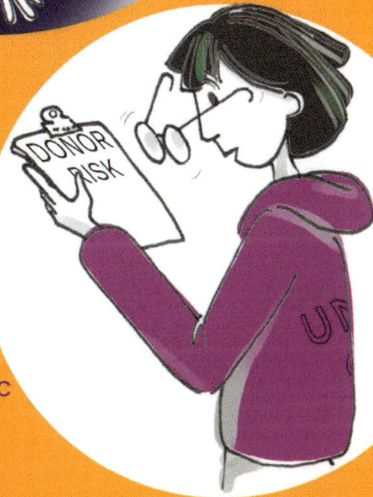

You can extract stem cells from your **BLOOD**, from **MILK TEETH**, or **ADIPOSE TISSUE** (in other words, **FAT**) - but there's a risk that these cells may already be damaged, or have undergone some sort of mutation in their adult life.

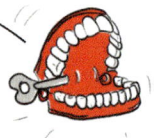

What we need is an untapped source of **perfectly formed** stem cells - one that is neither **painful** nor **invasive to access.**

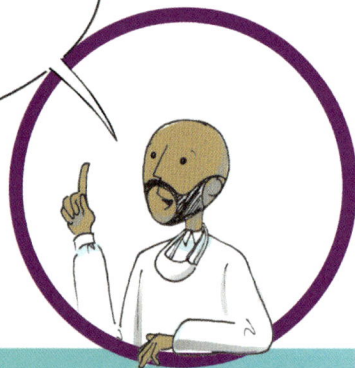

CORD BLOOD

At the point of birth, your stem cells are as close to **perfect** as they'll ever get.

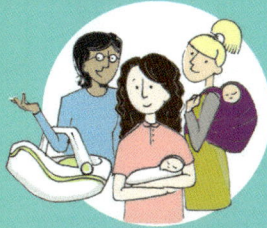

They're young, undamaged - and the **umbilical cord** is packed full of them.

The Maths is simple

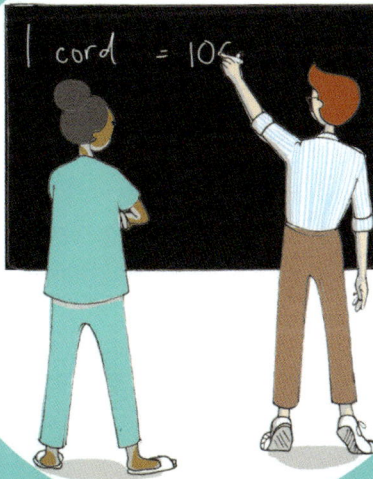

I cord = 100

One cord yields approximately **100ml of cord blood** - and that's enough for **one potentially life-saving transplant.**

WANT TO KNOW WHY ELSE IT'S "ALL ABOUT THE CORD?"

Approximately **680,000 births** are recorded each year in the UK - and whilst 25% of these will yield cords that are unsuitable, a staggering **510,000 umbilical cords** are still available.

The process is **non-invasive, non-painful** and **doesn't compromise childbirth.**

Umbilical cords currently go up in smoke as biological waste - keeping hold of them costs us **absolutely nothing.**

The cons?
There aren't any.

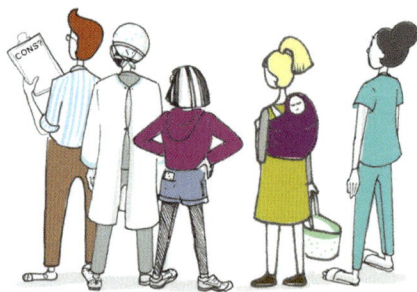

5

A VERY CLEVER STORAGE SOLUTION

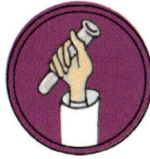

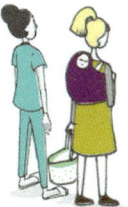

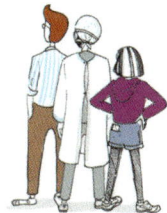

So, now we know WHICH stem cells to use, and we know WHERE to find them - how do we go about using them?

We freeze them.

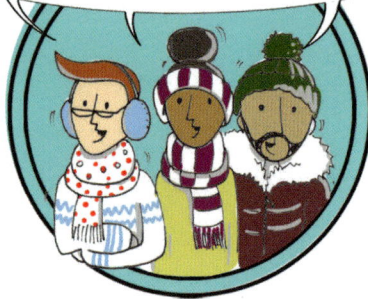

These uncorrupted, near-perfect cells are isolated, processed, and then popped into a cryogenic canister, which freezes them at approximately minus 180 degrees Celsius. This preserves their awesome, regenerating powers, meaning that they can be called upon, and replicated, when needed.

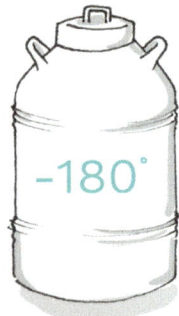

−180°

Better still, they can remain this way for over **100 years**.

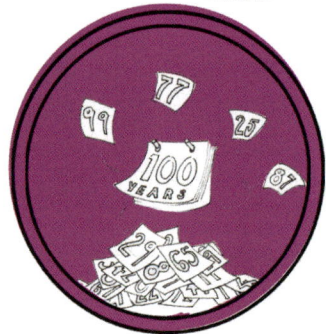

It's the ultimate life insurance.

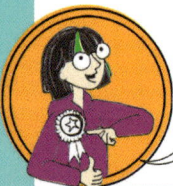

6

WHY YOU NEED A FAMILY BIO BANK

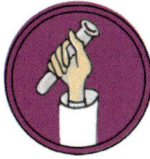

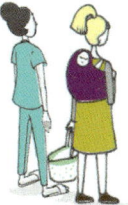

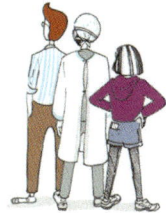

In an ideal world, we would all have our stem cells collected at the point of birth and frozen. In doing this, you would have also created a family 'bio-bank'.

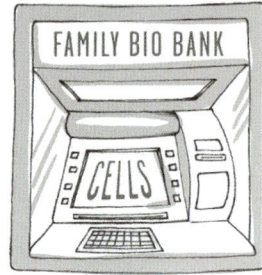

FAMILY BIO BANK
CELLS

Here's how it works:

You are a perfect match for your own stem cells (that part, at least, is obvious)

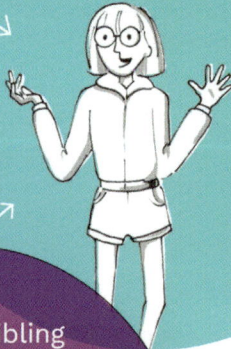

A parent has a 50% chance of being a stem cell match (a very good ratio)

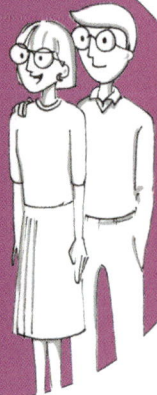

A sibling has a 25% chance of being a stem cell match (still a fighting chance)

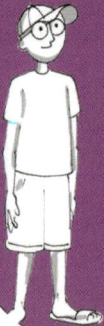

With a family bio-bank, there is no wait for treatment. Your stem cells or those of your child, or sibling, are immediately shipped, ready to be put to use

To put it into context, many patients in need of a life-saving operation spend several months waiting for a perfect stem cell match. If you are an ethnic minority, you may wait even longer. Most often, when a stem cell match cannot be found, it is imported from abroad,

costing upwards of 30,000 Euros.

And as more and more applications are made, the waiting list for a stem cell match becomes longer.

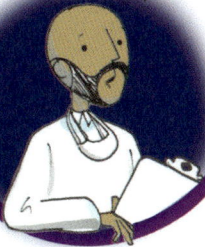

In some cases, by the time a match is found, it is too late.

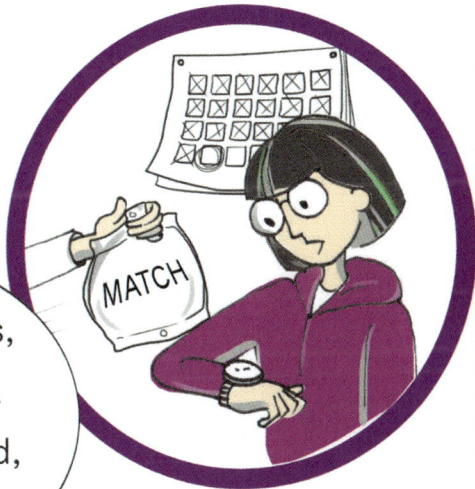

Which is why a

NATIONAL STEM CELL BANK

is also needed.

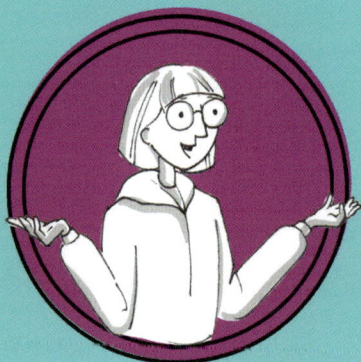

Which sounds **complicated**, but it's not.

All it takes is for more women to donate their cord at the point of birth.
The more cords are donated, the more stem cells we will bank.
And the more stem cells we bank, the greater the chances we have of finding a **match**.

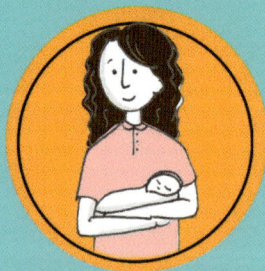

A NATIONAL BANK OF BRITISH STEM CELLS FOR BRITISH CITIZENS WOULD NOT ONLY SAVE COSTS, BUT IT WOULD SAVE LIVES.

IN FACT, FOR EVERY CORD DONATED, ONE LIFE CAN BE SAVED.

Each and every one of us, regardless of our age, ethnicity and wealth should have access to this.

7

BUT WHAT HAPPENS IF I GET ILL?

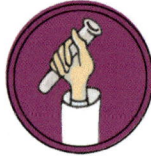

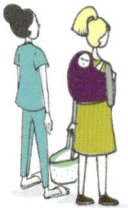

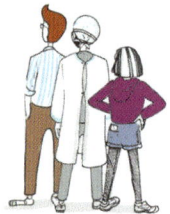

IT'S SIMPLE.

Your stem cells, or genetic match - taken from a well-stocked, ethically-diverse stem cell bank - are taken out of storage, transported to the hospital ready for the transplant, and injected into the site of damage or injury.

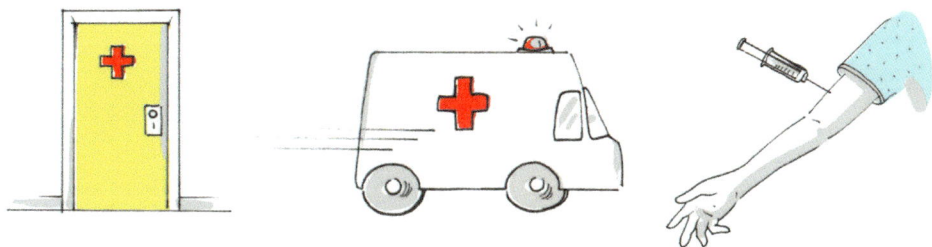

Once injected, they get to work - repairing, regenerating, and rejuvenating where they're needed. It's like resetting the software on your computer.

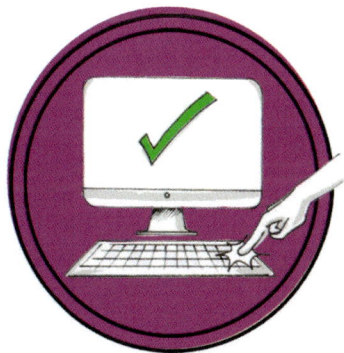

SO FAR,
82 DISEASES ARE TREATABLE USING STEM CELL THERAPY.

IN TEN YEARS TIME, WE SHOULD BE AIMING TO TREAT 820.

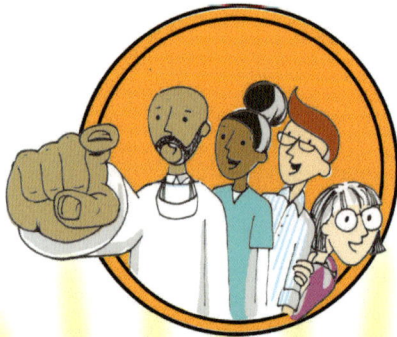

WHICH IS WHY WE NEED YOUR HELP.

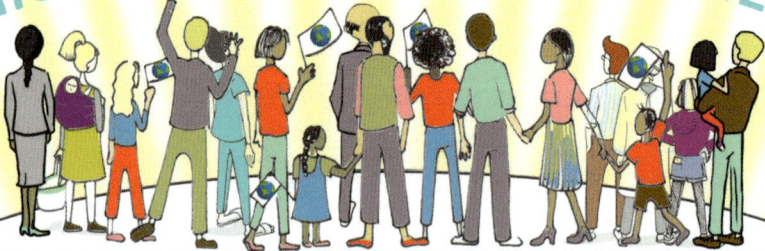

8

A BRAVE NEW WORLD

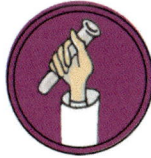

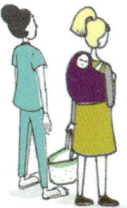

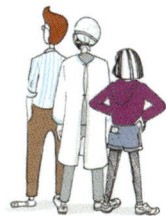

Today, more than ever before,
we're realising the staggering potential of
stem cell therapy.

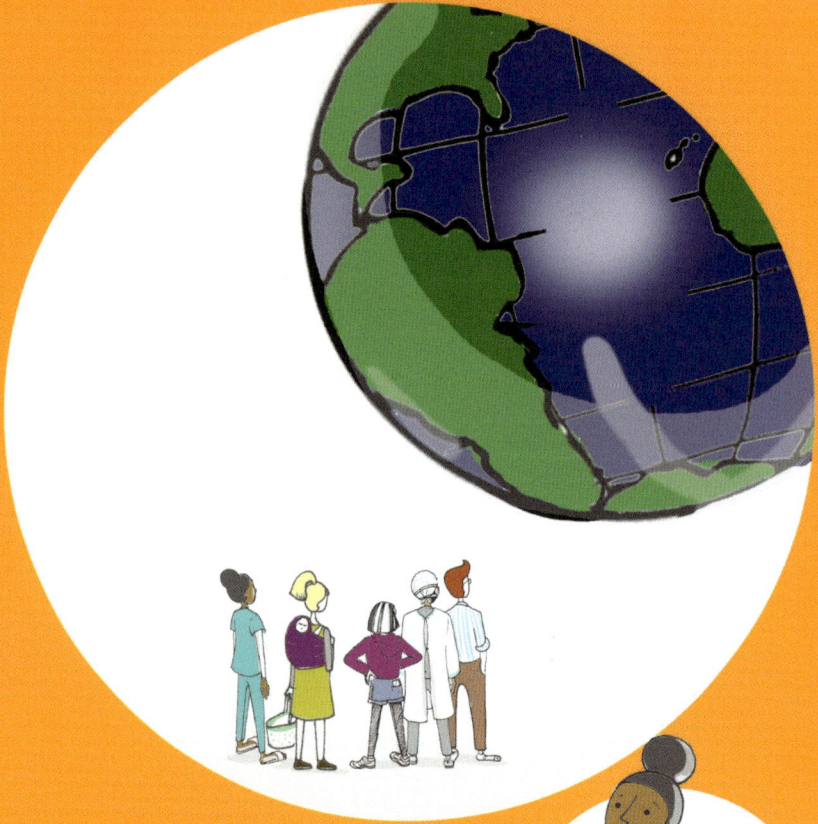

As our world becomes more
personalised, so too
does our medicine.

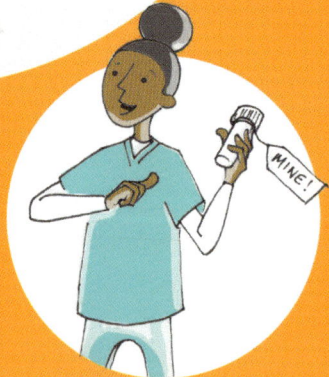

As physicists and researchers push for greater knowledge, so too do we.

As our understanding of stem cells grows, so too do studies into life-saving therapies.

Soon, conditions such as heart disease, brain disease, autism and strokes won't just be results on a piece of paper, they'll be treatable, curable diseaes.

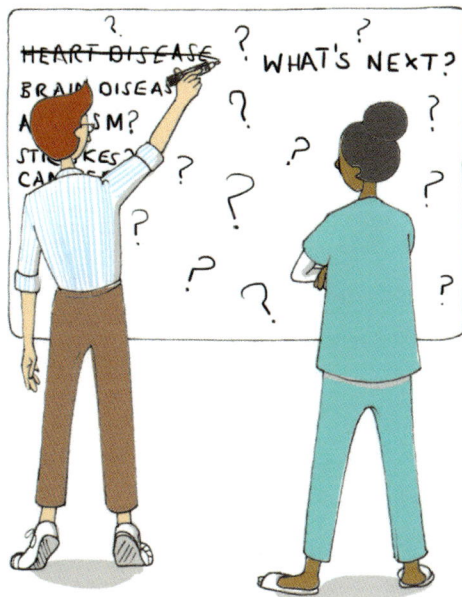

This is our future; and it's a bright one.

Only one question remains:

ARE YOU READY FOR IT?

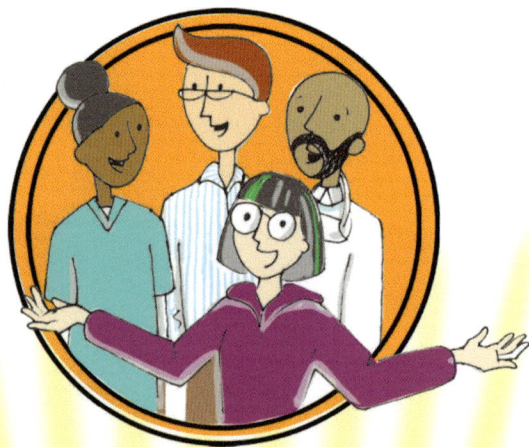

SO WHICH DISEASES CAN BE TREATED USING CORD BLOOD?

CANCERS

Acute lymphoblastic leukemia (ALL)
Acute myeloid leukemia (AML)
Burkitt's lymphoma
Chronic myeloid leukemia (CML)
Juvenile myelomonocytic leukemia (JMML)
Non-Hodgkin's lymphoma
Hodgkin's lymphoma
Lymphomatoid granulomatosis
Myelodysplastic syndrome (MDS)
Chronic myelomonocytic leukemia (CMML)
Bone Marrow Failure Syndromes
Amegakaryocytic thrombocytopenia
Autoimmune neutropenia (severe)
Congenital dyserythropoietic anemia
Cyclic neutropenia
Diamond-Blackfan anemia
Evan's syndrome
Fanconi anemia
Glanzmann's disease
Juvenile dermatomyositis
Kostmann's syndrome
Red cell aplasia
Shwachman syndrome
Severe aplastic anemia
Congenital sideroblastic anemia
Thrombocytopenia with absent radius (TAR syndrome)
Dyskeratosis congenita

BLOOD DISORDERS

Sickle-cell anemia (hemoglobin SS)
HbSC disease
Sickle βo Thalassemia
α-thalassemia major (hydrops fetalis)
β-thalassemia major (Cooley's anemia)
β-thalassemia intermedia
E-βo thalassemia
E-β+ thalassemia

METABOLIC DISORDERS
Adrenoleukodystrophy Gaucher's disease (infantile)
Metachromatic leukodystrophy
Krabbe disease (globoid cell leukodystrophy)
Gunther disease
Hermansky-Pudlak syndrome
Hurler syndrome
Hurler-Scheie syndrome
Hunter syndrome
Sanfilippo syndrome
Maroteaux-Lamy syndrome
Mucolipidosis Type II, III
Alpha mannosidosis
Niemann Pick Syndrome, type A and B
Sandhoff Syndrome
Tay-Sachs Disease
Lesch-Nyhan disease
Immunodeficiencies
Ataxia telangiectasia
Chronic granulomatous disease
DiGeorge syndrome
IKK gamma deficiency
Immune dysregulation polyendocrineopathy
X-linked Mucolipidosis, Type II
Myelokathexis X-linked immunodeficiency
Severe combined immunodeficiency
Adenosine deaminase deficiency
Wiskott-Aldrich syndrome
X-linked agammaglobulinemia
X-linked lymphoproliferative disease
Omenn's syndrome
Reticular dysplasia
Thymic dysplasia
Leukocyte adhesion deficiency

OTHER CONDITIONS
Osteopetrosis
Langerhans cell histiocytosis
Hemophargocytic lymphohistiocytosis

A HANDY GLOSSARY

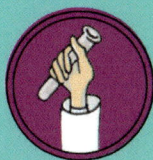

Adipose tissue - In other words, fat. This loose connective tissue contains adipocytes (fat cells), helping to insulate and cushion the body.

Bone marrow - The spongy tissue inside some of the bones in the body, including the hip and thigh bones. Bone marrow is a rich source of stem cells.

Cells - These are the structural units that make up a living organism, for example, the human body. Cells contain the necessary data for regulating function and transmitting information. They can change shape, mutate, and produce identical copies of themselves. The human body contains more than 30 trillion cells.

Cord blood - Blood found in the umbilical cord. Cord blood is also present in the placenta, after birth, and is a rich source of stem cells.

Cord tissue - This is tissue from the umbilical cord. It contains powerful stem cells, which help to repair and rebuild.

Cryogenic canister - A medical container, which uses liquid nitrogen to freeze contents to minus 180 degrees Celsius.

Embryo - The earliest stage of development in a living organism. A human embryo is so called up to eight weeks from the point of fertilisation.

Foetus - A prenatal human, midway between embryo and birth. The term 'foetus' is used eight weeks from the point of fertilisation.

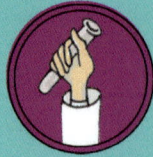

General anaesthetic - A medically-controlled state of unconsciousness, used to make a surgical procedure safer and more comfortable.

Organ - A collection of tissues, which combine to create a single, functional unit inside the body. The heart, liver, kidneys and lungs are just a few examples of an organ.

Placenta - An organ that connects the developing foetus to the uterine wall, providing oxygen and nutrients to growing babies whilst removing waste products. Also known as 'afterbirth'.

Regenerative medicine - A branch of medicine that supports the use of specialised cells, to help heal and repair previously irreparable tissue and organs in the body.

Stem cells - These are specialist cells, otherwise known as the 'building blocks of life'. Their role in the body is to multiply, to help replenish dying cells and regenerate damaged tissues.

Umbilical cord - A conduit between the foetus and the placenta, which supplies the foetus with oxygenated blood from the placenta. Otherwise known as the 'birth cord'.

Printed in Great Britain
by Amazon